let it flow

A Journal to Support You on Your Breastfeeding Journey

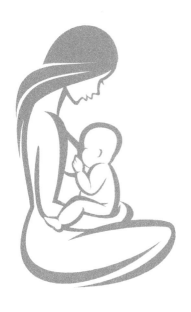

EMILY L. KENDALL

Copyright © 2023 by Emily Kendall. All rights reserved.

This book or any portion thereof may not be reproduced or used in any manner whatsoever without the express written permission of the publisher except for the use of brief quotations in a scholarly work or book review. For permissions or further information contact Braughler Books LLC at info@braughlerbooks.com.

The views and opinions expressed in this work are those of the author and do not necessarily reflect the views and opinions of Braughler Books LLC.

Stock photo images by Shutterstock

Printed in the United States of America

First Printing, 2023

ISBN 978-1-955791-69-4

Library of Congress Control Number: 2023916525

Ordering Information: Special discounts are available on quantity purchases by bookstores, corporations, associations, and others. For details, contact the publisher at sales@braughlerbooks.com or at 937-58-BOOKS.

For questions or comments about this book, please write to info@braughlerbooks.com.

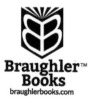

Mom

Baby

Date Started

I dedicate this journal to (it's okay to say yourself)

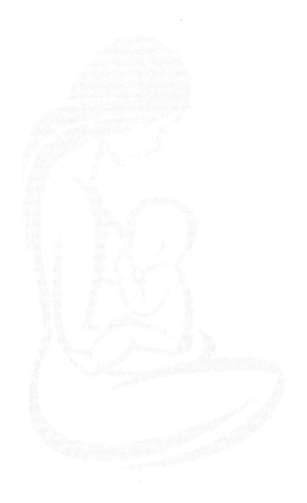

THE BIRTH OF THIS JOURNAL

Dear Friend,

You know those people who say, "Oh, I could have fed the whole hospital nursery!" or post pics of deep freezers crammed full of breastmilk storage bags? I am not one of those people. I am the person who would hide in my office hooked up to my pump for a "power pump" session - twenty on, ten off - and cringe at the resulting ¾ of an ounce. Total. Nothing quite picked at my deepest fear - *you are not good enough* - like the output from the pump.

I've had a long breastfeeding journey, starting with my first born who arrived at 29 weeks and two days. Direct breastfeeding wasn't an option for over a month. Even when we brought her home after two full months in the neonatal intensive care unit (NICU), I could only nurse her twice a day. I had to pump the rest and fortify with formula. My supply never had a chance, all it knew was the pump. I exhausted every resource, desperate to get it up. The teas, the supplements, the consultants, the warm compresses, warm showers, even dipping each boob in a bowl full of warm water. After 11 months, I hung up the pumping tubes. I shoved all my pumping gear up on the highest shelf in the darkest corner of the nursery closet.

Three years later, my son was born at 37 weeks and two days (well done, uterus). I latched him as soon as he slid out. Then the doctors and nurses took him and the room fell silent. We received an at birth diagnosis of Down syndrome. The details of that diagnosis delivery I will spare you for another book, just know he never lets anyone take our joy. As a result, we got booked on another tour through the NICU for a three week stay. The neonatologist asked if I planned to breastfeed him. When I responded in the affirmative, she scoffed, "don't expect much." I felt like saying, we clearly won't from you, but we will from him. Fortunately with the support of the wonderful NICU nurses and a supportive lactation staff we got off to a great start.

He was a champion breastfeeder, and I was able to nurse him more frequently. I still had to pump and fortify, and could never pump enough to replace a full feeding. This led me to the bowels of the internet, digging through the cited sources of a website called *www.kellymom.com*. Through this doom scrolling I learned a pre-pumping session technique that involved squeezing and releasing all of your muscles (mainly clenching my butt) and then massaging your boobs. This routine elicited some heavy and heartfelt sighs from my husband, but no increased supply.

By this point I was working four breast pumps: Ameda hospital grade upstairs in the nursery; Spectra S2 downstairs in the family room; Medela hospital grade at the office I begged HR to install; and the OG Medela Pump 'n Style in the minivan to bang out pumping sessions on my commute. After ten months, I packed all of that up, returned the Ameda and gave the Spectra to an expecting neighbor. I cleared out all the pump parts, filled our recycling bin with plastic flanges and slammed the lid. I had an IUD slid into place. DONE!

Ha. Nope. Four weeks shy of my 39th birthday, I found out I was pregnant, a 0.01% chance. By the grace of God this sweet girl arrived on her due date and immediately latched. We got sent home 24 hours later. I got to breastfeed her exclusively, a whole new experience. I felt like a first time, third time parent. Everything seemed to be working until our two month check-up. Her weight gain was not where it should have been. In an attempt to be helpful, the on-staff lactation consultant evaluated our latch, and suggested I had low supply and not enough mammary tissue to produce. I lost my shit. Completely fell apart. Failing. I was failing my child. I am a failure and I can't do this. *I am not good enough!* I was fully pulled under by that fear and the fear of having to return to the pump. My husband reassured me that the pediatrician didn't seem that concerned and wanted to see us back in a month.

After I pulled myself together, I stepped back and reflected. I also called in the Mary Poppins of lactation consultants. Wonderful and wise, she swept into the house with her special scale and weighed the baby before and after she ate. She confirmed what deep down I already knew - the latch and milk transfer were solid. We reviewed what had been happening the past month. The baby had a stuffy nose for two weeks. Our family experienced a stressful event related to my husband's business. I had been using a Haakaa pump on one side while

LET IT FLOW

feeding on the other, and was probably feeding the freezer instead. I made some adjustments and kept breastfeeding.

Even armed with that reassurance, I couldn't completely shake the fear. I religiously set my alarm every two hours to wake up and feed the baby. One night I overslept and four hours elapsed. I woke up and so did the narrative in my head. "You are a lazy piece of shit! I can't believe you overslept. You are failing the baby!" She was sleeping peacefully. My next thought - this has got to stop. I would never speak to my friends or family like this. I would never speak to anyone like this out loud, even if they were on my shit list and even if I really wanted to. So why am I talking like this to myself?

So, I started a journal practice. Everyday, ideally at the start of the day (honestly, when I remembered), I wrote down the following three things: something nice about myself, something I am grateful for, and what I call a "lactation visualization" to encourage let down (you know when you sort of need to pee and you hear or see water running and immediately have to pee - similar concept but with boobs and breastmilk). These visualizations usually included water and warmth, but did not involve dipping my nips into cereal bowls of warm water. That check up the next month? The baby's weight was right on track.

This journal practice allowed me to shift from fear to the present. From "not enough" to "it's okay". I became more aware of the running commentary in my head and started speaking more kindly to myself. I remembered to take myself less seriously and welcome the absurdity with a laugh. It helped me get into a calm and present state for feedings. It also helped me remember why I chose to breastfeed, and reflect back on why I busted my boobs to breastfeed my older two children. I loved and cherished the experience of breastfeeding. The sweet little hands cupped around my breast. The whispery eyelashes that slowly drop to rest on chubby cheeks towards the end of a feeding. The satisfying lip smack after pulling off. All of the warmth and the love that we get to exchange.

This journaling process made the daily marathon of breastfeeding a more fulfilling experience. I have been able to embrace the fullness of it - all its ups and downs, setbacks and clogged ducts - from a perspective of self-love and compassion. It helped me, and I am putting it out in the universe with the hope it will help someone else. Even if you just use it as a flat surface for your pump, I'll take that as a win.

With love to you and yours.
Let it flow –
Emily

{ 10 }

HOW TO USE THIS JOURNAL

Before getting started, please know that this journal process is something that I found helpful for me. I am not an expert, nor is this process based on extensive research. Heaven knows there is so much on social media from "experts" that even the Virgin Mary went dark on Insta. Please use this journal however it works for you. You can write in it once, do it everyday, do it sometimes, or like I said, use it as a flat surface to stabilize your pump. The point is - it's yours to make your own. Just like your nursing journey is yours to make your own. Here is how I designed this journal practice to work.

The prompts are the same everyday. I wanted something easy and low pressure that I could jot down quickly. I also wanted to build a habit, hence the repetition of the prompts. I wrote down different responses most days. Sometimes my responses were similar or the exact same, because like we all do, I have so much information to keep straight in my head.

Here are the prompts:

Something Nice About Myself

Give yourself a compliment like you would give a friend. This was often the hardest prompt for me. It's easy for me to say something nice about someone else. I'm in sales and marketing after all. It was not always easy for me to say something nice about myself. When I got stuck, I would imagine what my friends would say. This is a compliment you can return to when that mean girl voice starts harping in your ear. After doing this practice for a while, you have a whole host of nice things to say to yourself, and suddenly Regina George isn't so loud.

Something I am Grateful For

I love a good gratitude practice. Once I get going I can come up with so many things that fill my heart with gratitude. If I am really stuck I will channel my inner Julie Andrews and belt out "My Favorite Things." Unfortunately my inner channeling does not mean my voice sounds like hers and mostly I get eye rolls or moans from the bigger kids. For the purpose of this particular journal practice, I wanted to focus on one thing that was easy to think of and easy to remember. My espresso machine was a frequent mention under this prompt. As well as my anniversary edition soundtrack to *The Sound of Music*.

My Lactation Visualization

I started doing this to help encourage let down. Getting ready to nurse and get latched could get a little frantic for me - especially when the baby was fussing, the toddler was climbing on something he shouldn't and the six year old was blaring Bieber. I used this visual cue to settle down, settle in, take some deep breaths and hopefully encourage milk flow. I had the most fun with it and I encourage you to do the same. I would often visualize falling rain (even better when it was actually raining), the lull of ocean waves, or the first warm sips of my morning coffee.

Every two weeks there is space for a self check in - like a friend dropping in to see how you are doing. This is your space to reflect on how things are going and how you feel.

Most importantly, remember this is your breastfeeding journey and your journal. Let it flow.

LET IT FLOW

DATE

Something nice about myself:

Something I am grateful for:

Lactation Visualization:

LET IT FLOW

DATE

Something nice about myself:

Something I am grateful for:

Lactation Visualization:

LET IT FLOW

DATE

Something nice about myself:

Something I am grateful for:

Lactation Visualization:

{ 18 }

LET IT FLOW

DATE

Something nice about myself:

Something I am grateful for:

Lactation Visualization:

LET IT FLOW

DATE

Something nice about myself:

Something I am grateful for:

Lactation Visualization:

LET IT FLOW

DATE

Something nice about myself:

Something I am grateful for:

Lactation Visualization:

LET IT FLOW

DATE

Something nice about myself:

Something I am grateful for:

Lactation Visualization:

LET IT FLOW

DATE

Something nice about myself:

Something I am grateful for:

Lactation Visualization:

LET IT FLOW

DATE

Something nice about myself:

Something I am grateful for:

Lactation Visualization:

LET IT FLOW

DATE

Something nice about myself:

Something I am grateful for:

Lactation Visualization:

LET IT FLOW

DATE

Something nice about myself:

Something I am grateful for:

Lactation Visualization:

LET IT FLOW

DATE

Something nice about myself:

Something I am grateful for:

Lactation Visualization:

LET IT FLOW

DATE

Something nice about myself:

Something I am grateful for:

Lactation Visualization:

LET IT FLOW

DATE

Something nice about myself:

Something I am grateful for:

Lactation Visualization:

LET IT FLOW

CHECK-IN:

DATE

How am I doing?

LET IT FLOW

LET IT FLOW

DATE

Something nice about myself:

Something I am grateful for:

Lactation Visualization:

LET IT FLOW

DATE

Something nice about myself:

Something I am grateful for:

Lactation Visualization:

{ 33 }

LET IT FLOW

DATE

Something nice about myself:

Something I am grateful for:

Lactation Visualization:

LET IT FLOW

DATE

Something nice about myself:

Something I am grateful for:

Lactation Visualization:

LET IT FLOW

DATE

Something nice about myself:

Something I am grateful for:

Lactation Visualization:

LET IT FLOW

DATE

Something nice about myself:

Something I am grateful for:

Lactation Visualization:

LET IT FLOW

DATE

Something nice about myself:

Something I am grateful for:

Lactation Visualization:

LET IT FLOW

DATE

Something nice about myself:

Something I am grateful for:

Lactation Visualization:

LET IT FLOW

DATE

Something nice about myself:

Something I am grateful for:

Lactation Visualization:

LET IT FLOW

DATE

Something nice about myself:

Something I am grateful for:

Lactation Visualization:

LET IT FLOW

DATE

Something nice about myself:

Something I am grateful for:

Lactation Visualization:

LET IT FLOW

DATE

Something nice about myself:

Something I am grateful for:

Lactation Visualization:

LET IT FLOW

DATE

Something nice about myself:

Something I am grateful for:

Lactation Visualization:

LET IT FLOW

DATE

Something nice about myself:

Something I am grateful for:

Lactation Visualization:

LET IT FLOW

CHECK-IN:

DATE

How am I doing?

LET IT FLOW

LET IT FLOW

DATE

Something nice about myself:

Something I am grateful for:

Lactation Visualization:

LET IT FLOW

DATE

Something nice about myself:

Something I am grateful for:

Lactation Visualization:

LET IT FLOW

DATE

Something nice about myself:

Something I am grateful for:

Lactation Visualization:

LET IT FLOW

DATE

Something nice about myself:

Something I am grateful for:

Lactation Visualization:

LET IT FLOW

DATE

Something nice about myself:

Something I am grateful for:

Lactation Visualization:

LET IT FLOW

DATE

Something nice about myself:

Something I am grateful for:

Lactation Visualization:

LET IT FLOW

DATE

Something nice about myself:

Something I am grateful for:

Lactation Visualization:

LET IT FLOW

DATE

Something nice about myself:

Something I am grateful for:

Lactation Visualization:

LET IT FLOW

DATE

Something nice about myself:

Something I am grateful for:

Lactation Visualization:

LET IT FLOW

DATE

Something nice about myself:

Something I am grateful for:

Lactation Visualization:

LET IT FLOW

DATE

Something nice about myself:

Something I am grateful for:

Lactation Visualization:

LET IT FLOW

DATE

Something nice about myself:

Something I am grateful for:

Lactation Visualization:

LET IT FLOW

DATE

Something nice about myself:

Something I am grateful for:

Lactation Visualization:

LET IT FLOW

DATE

Something nice about myself:

Something I am grateful for:

Lactation Visualization:

LET IT FLOW

CHECK-IN:

DATE

How am I doing?

LET IT FLOW

LET IT FLOW

DATE

Something nice about myself:

Something I am grateful for:

Lactation Visualization:

LET IT FLOW

DATE

Something nice about myself:

Something I am grateful for:

Lactation Visualization:

LET IT FLOW

DATE

Something nice about myself:

Something I am grateful for:

Lactation Visualization:

LET IT FLOW

DATE

Something nice about myself:

Something I am grateful for:

Lactation Visualization:

LET IT FLOW

DATE

Something nice about myself:

Something I am grateful for:

Lactation Visualization:

LET IT FLOW

DATE

Something nice about myself:

Something I am grateful for:

Lactation Visualization:

LET IT FLOW

DATE

Something nice about myself:

Something I am grateful for:

Lactation Visualization:

LET IT FLOW

DATE

Something nice about myself:

Something I am grateful for:

Lactation Visualization:

{ 73 }

LET IT FLOW

DATE

Something nice about myself:

Something I am grateful for:

Lactation Visualization:

LET IT FLOW

DATE

Something nice about myself:

Something I am grateful for:

Lactation Visualization:

LET IT FLOW

DATE

Something nice about myself:

Something I am grateful for:

Lactation Visualization:

LET IT FLOW

DATE

Something nice about myself:

Something I am grateful for:

Lactation Visualization:

LET IT FLOW

DATE

Something nice about myself:

Something I am grateful for:

Lactation Visualization:

LET IT FLOW

DATE

Something nice about myself:

Something I am grateful for:

Lactation Visualization:

LET IT FLOW

CHECK-IN:

DATE

How am I doing?

LET IT FLOW

LET IT FLOW

DATE

Something nice about myself:

Something I am grateful for:

Lactation Visualization:

LET IT FLOW

DATE

Something nice about myself:

Something I am grateful for:

Lactation Visualization:

LET IT FLOW

DATE

Something nice about myself:

Something I am grateful for:

Lactation Visualization:

LET IT FLOW

DATE

Something nice about myself:

Something I am grateful for:

Lactation Visualization:

LET IT FLOW

DATE

Something nice about myself:

Something I am grateful for:

Lactation Visualization:

LET IT FLOW

DATE

Something nice about myself:

Something I am grateful for:

Lactation Visualization:

LET IT FLOW

DATE

Something nice about myself:

Something I am grateful for:

Lactation Visualization:

LET IT FLOW

DATE

Something nice about myself:

Something I am grateful for:

Lactation Visualization:

LET IT FLOW

DATE

Something nice about myself:

Something I am grateful for:

Lactation Visualization:

LET IT FLOW

DATE

Something nice about myself:

Something I am grateful for:

Lactation Visualization:

LET IT FLOW

DATE

Something nice about myself:

Something I am grateful for:

Lactation Visualization:

LET IT FLOW

DATE

Something nice about myself:

Something I am grateful for:

Lactation Visualization:

LET IT FLOW

DATE

Something nice about myself:

Something I am grateful for:

Lactation Visualization:

LET IT FLOW

DATE

Something nice about myself:

Something I am grateful for:

Lactation Visualization:

LET IT FLOW

CHECK-IN:

DATE

How am I doing?

LET IT FLOW

LET IT FLOW

DATE

Something nice about myself:

Something I am grateful for:

Lactation Visualization:

LET IT FLOW

DATE

Something nice about myself:

Something I am grateful for:

Lactation Visualization:

LET IT FLOW

DATE

Something nice about myself:

Something I am grateful for:

Lactation Visualization:

LET IT FLOW

DATE

Something nice about myself:

Something I am grateful for:

Lactation Visualization:

LET IT FLOW

DATE

Something nice about myself:

Something I am grateful for:

Lactation Visualization:

LET IT FLOW

DATE

Something nice about myself:

Something I am grateful for:

Lactation Visualization:

LET IT FLOW

DATE

Something nice about myself:

Something I am grateful for:

Lactation Visualization:

LET IT FLOW

DATE

Something nice about myself:

Something I am grateful for:

Lactation Visualization:

LET IT FLOW

DATE

Something nice about myself:

Something I am grateful for:

Lactation Visualization:

LET IT FLOW

DATE

Something nice about myself:

Something I am grateful for:

Lactation Visualization:

LET IT FLOW

DATE

Something nice about myself:

Something I am grateful for:

Lactation Visualization:

LET IT FLOW

DATE

Something nice about myself:

Something I am grateful for:

Lactation Visualization:

LET IT FLOW

DATE

Something nice about myself:

Something I am grateful for:

Lactation Visualization:

LET IT FLOW

DATE

Something nice about myself:

Something I am grateful for:

Lactation Visualization:

LET IT FLOW

CHECK-IN:

DATE

How am I doing?

LET IT FLOW

LET IT FLOW

DATE

Something nice about myself:

Something I am grateful for:

Lactation Visualization:

LET IT FLOW

DATE

Something nice about myself:

Something I am grateful for:

Lactation Visualization:

LET IT FLOW

DATE

Something nice about myself:

Something I am grateful for:

Lactation Visualization:

LET IT FLOW

DATE

Something nice about myself:

Something I am grateful for:

Lactation Visualization:

LET IT FLOW

DATE

Something nice about myself:

Something I am grateful for:

Lactation Visualization:

LET IT FLOW

DATE

Something nice about myself:

Something I am grateful for:

Lactation Visualization:

LET IT FLOW

DATE

Something nice about myself:

Something I am grateful for:

Lactation Visualization:

LET IT FLOW

DATE

Something nice about myself:

Something I am grateful for:

Lactation Visualization:

LET IT FLOW

DATE

Something nice about myself:

Something I am grateful for:

Lactation Visualization:

LET IT FLOW

DATE

Something nice about myself:

Something I am grateful for:

Lactation Visualization:

LET IT FLOW

DATE

Something nice about myself:

Something I am grateful for:

Lactation Visualization:

LET IT FLOW

DATE

Something nice about myself:

Something I am grateful for:

Lactation Visualization:

LET IT FLOW

DATE

Something nice about myself:

Something I am grateful for:

Lactation Visualization:

LET IT FLOW

DATE

Something nice about myself:

Something I am grateful for:

Lactation Visualization:

LET IT FLOW

CHECK-IN:

DATE

How am I doing?

LET IT FLOW

LET IT FLOW

DATE

Something nice about myself:

Something I am grateful for:

Lactation Visualization:

LET IT FLOW

DATE

Something nice about myself:

Something I am grateful for:

Lactation Visualization:

LET IT FLOW

DATE

Something nice about myself:

Something I am grateful for:

Lactation Visualization:

LET IT FLOW

DATE

Something nice about myself:

Something I am grateful for:

Lactation Visualization:

LET IT FLOW

DATE

Something nice about myself:

Something I am grateful for:

Lactation Visualization:

LET IT FLOW

DATE

Something nice about myself:

Something I am grateful for:

Lactation Visualization:

{ 139 }

LET IT FLOW

DATE

Something nice about myself:

Something I am grateful for:

Lactation Visualization:

LET IT FLOW

DATE

Something nice about myself:

Something I am grateful for:

Lactation Visualization:

{ 141 }

LET IT FLOW

DATE

Something nice about myself:

Something I am grateful for:

Lactation Visualization:

LET IT FLOW

DATE

Something nice about myself:

Something I am grateful for:

Lactation Visualization:

LET IT FLOW

DATE

Something nice about myself:

Something I am grateful for:

Lactation Visualization:

LET IT FLOW

DATE

Something nice about myself:

Something I am grateful for:

Lactation Visualization:

LET IT FLOW

DATE

Something nice about myself:

Something I am grateful for:

Lactation Visualization:

LET IT FLOW

DATE

Something nice about myself:

Something I am grateful for:

Lactation Visualization:

LET IT FLOW

CHECK-IN:

DATE

How am I doing?

LET IT FLOW

LET IT FLOW

LET IT FLOW

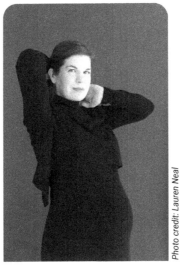
Photo credit: Lauren Neal

I'm an omni-mom - step-mom, mom of three, dog mom married to an awesome man and life partner. My oldest daughter was born at 29 weeks and two days and spent two months in the NICU. My son was diagnosed at birth with Down syndrome and spent three weeks in the NICU. I got pregnant with an IUD – a 0.01% chance – and welcomed another daughter in 2022 (if you have an IUD and you're reading this, I'm your statistic – so I've probably got you covered).

    I pumped and breastfed with my first two, and exclusively breastfed my third. I created this journaling process for myself to help find some peace and relieve the pressure and stress that can surround feeding. It has been a gift that I want to share. In exchange, I welcome the opportunity to connect with you. Please visit me at www.emilyLkendall.com.

Printed in the USA
CPSIA information can be obtained
at www.ICGtesting.com
LVHW052314271023
762325LV00017B/502